WHAT A PCP SHOULD EXPECT FROM A SPECIALIST

BANJI AWOSIKA

PREFACE

My name is Banji Awosika. My father and every one of his siblings had hypertension. At the time i was deciding my career path, he had lost a sibling due to complications of hypertension. I had always known I wanted to help people, as did my dad and due to my academic quests, he saw the potential for me to become a doctor. After a few years in med school, I left for a year to improve my financial situation. I went to work in London, UK as a cab driver. I actually fell in love with medicine and after I left it for a while, I realized I was actually in love with medicine. I missed it so much and realized that this was what I was called to do. Taking care and servicing the needs that people have, educating people and showing them how to get healthier. Lessening and eventually eliminating the need for medication became a very overwhelming passion for me over the years. The most rewarding aspect is hearing from the families of the patients that I have taken care of and seeing the impact on their lives as well as their kids. When the mother of a patient comes back and tells me they lost ten pounds and they are off medications. That blesses the socks off of me. The whole idea is to create ambassadors of this message from patients to the staff, to the families of the staff, to the families of the patients and this way it goes viral. That is really the impact I want to have. In order to do this, it is very important to be able to communicate with primary care physicians that see the patients and are in charge of their care. This book is for the caring primary care physician, who embraces the holistic approach to care given by a specialist and appreciates specialist feedback. For those who want to solve the problem of getting late feedback and communication from specialists who do not accept all insurances and do not encourage patients to follow-up with their primary care physician. Let's get started.

Banji Awosika 26-Sept-2016

TABLE OF CONTENTS

PREFACE i
TABLE OF CONTENTS ii
CHAPTER ONE
How quickly would you be able to see my patient 1
CHAPTER TWO
Do you take all insurances 4
CHAPTER THREE
Do you provide comprehensive one stop care for our patients...................................... 7
CHAPTER FOUR
Will I receive correspondence from you in a timely manner 10
CHAPTER FIVE
Patients not following up with primary care physician after seeing a specialist 13
CHAPTER SIX
Are your office staff members easy to work with 16
CHAPTER SEVEN
I can take care of the patients until they are close to requiring dialysis 20
ENDING CHAPTER

CHAPTER ONE

How quickly would you be able to see my patient

We aim to see patients within the same week, preferably within 48 hours

When the referral is received, the patient is scheduled at the next available appointment. We try to make this within 48 hours which usually is the case, but definitely within the week. This patient can be seen within 24 hours if need be. In this case, the primary care physician calling us, doctor to doctor, will be a plus but not a must. We tend to be quite flexible with the ultimate aim being to keep the patient out of the hospital. So, we tend to accommodate patients being seen at a moment's notice in order to achieve this goal.

The patient can be seen the same day if the specialist is called by the PCP. Again, as noted above, the patient can be seen the same day and the PCP call is a plus but it is not a must. The patient can be seen regardless of accompanying correspondence. This means although it is great to have notes from the PCP, lab work from the PCP and any radiological test that have been done, this is not a pre-requisite and the patient can be seen whether or not this information is available. Again, the goal here is to avoid the patient being admitted, so we want to see the patient at a moment's notice and initiate management of the patient to keep him out of the hospital and guide them onto a path towards great health. Now, depending on the acuity, the patient can actually be fast-tracked on that same day. So not only will we see the patient the same day, we could possibly see the patient immediately ahead of patients that have already been scheduled in the clinic.

To see patients quicker, our front desk staff gets patients scheduled. Once we receive a referral, the front desk staff actually call the patient. This way, the scheduling does not depend on the patient contacting us. Because once we get the referral from the PCP, we proceed immediately to contact the patients to get them scheduled as soon as possible. When the patient is scheduled, we then communicate with the PCP office to make them aware of the fact that the patient has been scheduled. The front desk will communicate with the PCP, with the primary care physician office to implement the completion of the checklist of required accompanying correspondence to improve the patient's care experience and the diagnostic capacity at the very first visit. Ongoing office visit reminders are done by the front desk.

We see patients whether or not other accompanying documentation is available

As already noted, we do see patients whether or not they have accompanying correspondence. In order to avoid admission and provide prompt service, patients may be seen without these accompanying correspondence. In this case, in-house investigations will be done including lab work, ultrasounds if needed, as this has a very quick turnaround for us. The primary care physician will be called regarding the management of this patient, again in a bid to prevent the patient from being admitted.

If the patient can make it to our office on any day between Monday and Thursday before the office closes, the patient will be seen

As already discussed and will be reiterated several times during this book, prevention of admission of the patient is one of our core missions. So the patient will be seen if he or she comes to the office while the office is open, on Mondays through to Thursdays. If patients come in late for their appointment, they will still be seen. However, they do tend to have to wait for the scheduled patients to be seen until there is an opening but they will be seen. Occasionally, when patients come in we also have the ability to provide a teleconference where they are seen by the physician who is at a remote location, again in a bid to prevent the patient from being admitted to the hospital.

On occasions, transportation is provided for patients

For patients that receive sedation usually during our vascular procedures, transportation may be provided if they do not have family support to transport them to and from the vascular clinic. Transportation can be arranged with Links services for other patients. Transportation other than Links may be provided as a courtesy if we are able to justify this as something above if they are going to be receiving sedation or if they have absolutely no means of arriving at the destination because of varying emergent situations, we do provide transportation for these patients.

The patient leaving hospital is given a priority

Post-hospitalization patients are seen as priorities for us, they are typically seen within a week of being discharged from the hospital to avoid re-admission. Sometimes they are seen within a couple of days, depending on their status upon discharge. Communication with patients is very frequent upon their discharge and they are actually called by our front desk staff to schedule their appointment for follow-up and depending on the situation, they may be seen on the same day or the next day but definitely within a week of discharge. Medication reconciliation is very important to these patients and re-evaluating their most current lab work upon discharge and at the time of visit becomes very important. This is the end of chapter one. In the next chapter we are going to be discussing insurances.

CHAPTER TWO

Do you take all insurances

Any health insurances we find that we are not on, we GET on

We have a very dedicated credential team and the heart of our providers is to be able to see every patient sent to us and impact the patient and their families. The responsibility level of the MD is very high, which means we take it upon ourselves to make sure the patient is seen and impacted. In order to do this, it is very important that we are on every insurance panel available so that every patient that is referred to us can and will be seen. We have a great track record and I have essentially never been denied by an insurance company to be on their panel of providers.

Great affordable plans for no-insurance patients

Healthcare in America is such that not everyone can afford insurance and not everyone opts to have an insurance for one reason or the other. We offer a great package for patients that have no insurance and there are actually repayment schedules available to these patients who can't afford to pay in one instalment. The tests may be included in the package or if the patients prefer or cannot afford this, will not be included in the package.

We tend to work within the request of the primary care physician as regards to the frequency of the office visit

With medical insurance being the way it is, United States officially capitated payments. We encourage the primary care physician to dictate the frequency of the office visit patients with us. With this, certain patients are seen less frequently and in the interim, we may draw lab work and follow the patient remotely if we find the patient to be stable enough for this. At times however, patients need to be seen more frequently because of acuity of their condition and in this case, we communicate with the primary care physician regarding this prior to seeing them. Remember, the mission here is to prevent the patient from being admitted to the hospital.

Creative ways to maintain convenience of the patient despite the insurance

As noted above, we strive to maintain convenience of the patient, as well as honoring the request of the primary care physician in regards to office visits by the patients with us the specialist. We also strive to avoid higher costed treatments. For example, intravenous iron is much more costly than oral iron. We discuss this with the primary care physician prior to initiating this treatment and since oral iron may actually work, although it would take much longer and after a prolonged period of time may still work very inefficiently. Sometimes this is the only option we have to treat the patient and this is done. Lab work is done in-house by other labs, outside labs, that accept their insurance when there are insurances that do not accept us as lab work providers. This is still done in-house for the convenience of the patient. At times, when we are unable to obtain an authorization to see the patient, we still provide as much guidance as we can over the phone or email and occasionally, by still seeing the patients without charging if need be.

Billing and coding specialists, insurance regulations compliance

Insurance rules and regulations are constantly changing. We have a dedicated biller and coder for this very dynamic problem here. Compliance is generally a very high priority for us and remaining in compliance is something we strive to do all the time. As a result of our in-depth knowledge of this, we communicate with the primary care physician officers, helping them to stay abreast if they are not already abreast themselves.

Prescription medications given based on insurance

Many disease entities can be treated effectively by more than one choice of medications. Preferably the choice of medication used should be based on clinical judgement, this is unfortunately not the case in several instances. Based on one's insurance, medication choices are categorized into levels or tiers of preference. As physicians we have to be stronger advocates for our patients and dialogue with the insurance companies with more intention so as to provide the care our patients need based on our clinical judgement and not the dictation of insurance. As a specialist the list of medications I utilize is shorter than that of my Primary care colleagues and as a result, I tend to go above and beyond to ensure my patients get the medication I feel the clinical scenario dictates. Based on prices, I also work closely with the pharmacists to ensure the medication is covered. E-prescribing also ensures great communication, reducing errors to the barest minimum. We are able to provide samples until there is clarity of the drugs that are actually covered by their insurance

No discrimination based on insurance

In our office, all patients are seen without the doctor being privy to patient's type of insurance until their chart is actually in front of them as they meet the patient and our policy simply demands all patient s to be seen regardless of their insurance as long as the visit is authorized by the insurance company. Essentially all patients have an equal opportunity to benefit from our care. The front desk and the doctors have zero discussion regarding type of insurance patient has.

The doctor provides care strictly based on acuity of disease and clinical judgement and not type of insurance

CHAPTER THREE

Do you provide comprehensive one stop care for our patients

Ability to diagnose mostly without referring to other facilities

A very important part of our patient management is in obtaining the correct diagnosis in a timely cost-efficient manner. We are able to do this as a result of :

- In-house laboratory where we perform all our test, with very few actually sent out
- In-house ultrasound which are very quickly read and interpreted by the physicians
- In-house vascular lab to very quickly diagnose and appropriately manage our patients tha require dialysis, initiating dialysis without putting them in the hospital
- In-house dialysis unit able to ensure patients are assessed and managed quickly eliminating the need for frequent visits of patients to the emergency room.

Avoid admitting patients into the hospital

We are able to avoid admitting patients because we are able to provide intravenous iron infusions which can be given every day. We typically give a total of ten IV, intravenous iron infusions over as quickly as ten days or depending on the convenience of the patient as infrequently as once a week for ten weeks. We are also able to give intramuscular injections of the Erythropoeitin stimulating agents. Patients requiring dialysis care can be given urgent hemodialysis sessions to avoid admissions to the hospital which is the most common reason why patients of dialysis are admitted to the hospital. The second most common reason for why patients are admitted to the hospital are for vascular access dysfunction and other issues which can also be managed appropriately in our vascular lab and outpatient. We are also able to administer intravenous Lasix to patients not on dialysis that are in our clinics to avoid admission to the hospital. We also are able to give subcutaneous Acthar as part of the treatment for glomerulonephritis.

These therapies when given are substantially cheaper than when given in the hospital, even after removing the cost of the hospital stay.

Able to see patients daily if need be for acute care

As a result of having multiple clinics and clinics on a daily basis Monday to Thursday, we are able to see patients as frequently- as they need to be seen. Sometimes, this is actually a daily visit to avoid a hospital admission and of course, communication is made with the primary care physician before this is done. Remember as I said several times and I will probably say it many more times, the goal and the mission is to avoid patients being admitted to the hospital. Lab work done in-house with its quick turn-around time guides their care which is why we are able to do this in the out-patient setting. Sometimes IV iron as mentioned above, intravenous iron, is given on a daily basis for ten days to avoid the patient from being admitted and to obtain improvement in their symptoms quicker.

Patients made aware of side-by-side care with the primary care physician

In order to provide optimal care, obtaining the trust of the patient is very important. We do this by our endorsement of the primary care physician that the patient already has put their trust in, as well as by endorsement by the primary care physician. Patient's confidence is boosted knowing the primary care physician is the best for his or her care. We do this by inviting the patient to conference with ourselves and the primary care physician so we are able to brainstorm their optimal management plan at the time of their office visit.

Communication with patients goes way beyond their office visit

Rapport with the office staff is very important i.e. rapport between office staff and the patient. For example, it is not uncommon for the other staff to visit the patients while they are in the hospital for whatever reason. There is 24-hour access to our care. There is always someone on call and available to speak to any physician that has not been seen by the practice. Email correspondence is also available for correspondence 24 hours a day. We also conference call, made wellness coach on a regular basis and newsletters are sent out monthly to keep educating the patient.

Multipronged education

Being seen by different physicians at different office visits is a system we use to increase accountability of the providers where they remain accountable to each other as they follow up on each other's patients. They are able to constructively critique the care given at their last visit, opening debate with one another for the best evidence-based approach to the care of the patient. We are able to reiterate things that were said and if necessary, clarify things said by the provider or ask the provider to come back and clarify if need be. There is also a recap of the plan of care at check-out by the front desk staff. There is also education by our lifestyle coach done in various formats including monthly newsletters. The patient also get educated by the TV contents shown in the patient lounge while they spend no more than a few minutes waiting to be roomed.

Ability to see the patient on the same day

We have a great office system with high capacity to see patients. This is made possible by our frequent clinics done daily, in the AM and in the PM for the convenience patients. Primary care physician making available correspondence regarding the patient is always a plus but patient

will be seen regardless of the availability of this correspondence. As long as the patient arrives before the close of office, the patient will be seen between Mondays and through Thursdays.

This brings us to the end of chapter three. Next, I will be discussing the receiving of correspondence, in a timely manner.

CHAPTER FOUR

Will I receive correspondence from you in a timely manner

Correspondence occurs before patient leaves exam room

Because of advanced technology, we have the ability to have notes faxed over to the primary care physician before the patient actually leaves the examination room. We have a scribing system which ensures that the progress note is done before a patient leaves the room. We allow some time for a possible conference with the primary care physician and the patient after the primary care physician receives the note. With Eprescribe, we are also able to have the prescription emailed to the pharmacy before the patient leaves. So the patient leaves the clinic and picks up the prescription right away.

Big changes

If there are big changes, we will call you with correspondence in front of you to discuss. To ensure collaborative care, we call the primary care physician in order to ensure that we are able to create an environment for the optimal management of the patient. Depending on acuity of care, the primary care physician will be called by the specialist while the patient is in the clinic. To brainstorm with the primary care physician regarding major changes, we hold the calls as a very high priority. In addition to this, non-nephrology issues thought to be important would also result in a call being made.

The patient won't be seen again unless either seen by the primary care physician or discussed with the primary care physician

To ensure proper correspondence, a call will be made to PCP prior to repeat office visits if there has not been any correspondence from his primary care physician. If the patient has not seen a primary care physician, we will strongly encourage an attempt to schedule an appointment while the patient is there. It will be made clear to the patient that a collaborative approach with the primary care physician leading the charge is strongly preferred for his care, making him realize that our ultimate mission of keeping the patient out of the hospital is actually more likely to succeed if the primary care physician is heading the charge.

We send notes and if required, labs to the primary care physician

Notes, progress notes are sent while the patient is in the room as has already been stated. If the primary care physician orders lab work to be done, this lab work is either sent with the progress notes or sometimes even before, depending on when the request for the labs were received. If requested by the patient, lab results are sent with the notes to the primary care physician. The patient also always gets a copy of his or her lab report after discussions with the patient.

Correspondence will go beyond office visit note.

Education for us is a very high priority. Regular newsletters will be mailed out ever so often, and these are designed in such a way to give the primary care physician an edge. Newsletters are made available for not only the primary care physician and his staff, but also for the patients in the primary care physician's office. Placing it in the patient lobby will be very beneficial both to the patient and to the primary care physician, as well as to us. It is a win-win-win situation. In the near future, CME dinners will also be made available, all in a bid to educate the patient and educate and be educated by the primary care physician, as there will be lots of dialogue during these meetings.

Direct access to me, the specialist, by cell 24 hours a day

My cellphone is made available to primary care physicians for direct access 24 hours a day. If I am with a patient, it will be answered by a scribe and the call will be returned before the end of the day. If a more urgent call back is needed, I suggest that a call back number be given. There is always someone on call, so if I am not on call, I am still available by my cell, but another doctor may be reached through the office.

I would offer to have office correspondence made easier

Office correspondence can be made easier with referral pads where our details are on the referral pad and the primary care physician just fills this out and faxes it. Once the patient is scheduled, the primary care physician office is notified. Newsletters in the patient lobby with call to action and should be placed as well. There will also be a trifold with our services clearly indicated all in a bid to make office correspondence and referrals much easier.

This brings us to the end of this chapter. In the next chapter, we will be discussing patients not following up with primary care physicians after seeing a specialist.

CHAPTER FIVE

Patients not following up with primary care physician after seeing a specialist

The patient will not be seen until he follows up with the primary care physician or until we discuss with the primary care physician

The patient will be strongly advised to see a primary care physician while he is in the office. In fact, we will endeavor to schedule an appointment with the primary care physician while the patient is in the office. We would also call the primary care physician to discuss before seeing.

Education of patient

It is very important to flow power to the primary care physician. The patient needs to understand that the primary care physician leads the charge. A well-visit is actually preferred to a sick-visit to the primary care physician and this will be clearly communicated to the patient.

No filling of prescription other than nephrology medications

The refill medications we prescribe is the ideal plan as opposed to refilling medications prescribed by other physicians. We tend to avoid prescribing any non-nephrology medications. That means we will prescribe blood pressure medications, vitamin D, any electrolytes imbalance supplementation or neutralization. We encourage patients to have all the medications they need to be prescribed, handled by the primary care physician that day and we actually offer to call the primary care physician for the patient.

Encourage wellness visits with primary care physicians

Patients are to be made aware and to understand that wellness visits are very important. This is part of the patient's education essentially letting the patient know that sick visits are more likely to have a favorable outcome if prior visits were wellness visits to the primary care physician. In essence, seeing the patients in his optimal state makes it easier and more optimal to treat him in his suboptimal state. Wellness visit with a clean bill of health is another feather in your cap. We also encourage the family of the patients to have their wellness visits with their primary care physician as soon as possible.

Flow power to primary care physician

We endeavor to make patients aware of the importance of the primary care physician. Various things are emphasized to the patient, especially in regards to the loyalty of the other patients that we take care of and how long they have been with him or her for. We describe in detail how well we work with the primary care physician and his office. We essentially endorse the primary care physician.

We schedule office visits to primary care physicians if patients have not been seen since our last encounter

Encouraging the patient to have a visit scheduled with his or her primary care physician while in our office is a high priority for us. Of course, we would have already discussed this with the primary care physician before seeing the patient, so we also give the patients an opportunity to actually speak with the primary care physician while in our office. We aim to eliminate any barriers to them visiting the primary care physician's office and this can also be overcome by the primary care physician with us flowing more power to him or her at that time. Telemedicine options can also be used in this situation to make for a more compelling effort to get the patient back into the primary care physician's office.

Communication with the primary care physician if the patient refuses to see the primary care physician anymore.

We find that it is important for the primary care physician to know if the patient is unhappy with his or her care. We encourage the patient to see the primary care physician and communicate their unhappiness giving the primary care physician a chance to rectify the situation. We strongly counsel the patient as to him or her entertaining the possibility of miscommunication and we also tend to further investigate if it was actually a primary care physician issue or the primary care physician's office as the actual issue, in which case we would advise the primary care physician accordingly.

This brings us to the end of chapter five. In the next chapter, we will be delving into the office staff being easy to work with for the primary care physician.

CHAPTER SIX

Are your office staff members easy to work with

Criteria for office staff for myself - they must be very easy to work with

My core values extend into my office environment. These core values are:
- Excellence
- Passion
- Respect
- Compassion
- Leadership
- Responsibility

The staff are chosen based on these core values. The staff are also trained based on these core values. The productivity bonus is very strongly influenced by their adhering to our core values.

Staff longevity with me is strongly influenced by feedback from patients

Clients are always right. Customer satisfaction is very important for us. Of course, as a business, customer acquisition is actually of greater importance but interestingly enough, customer acquisition drives customer satisfaction because we would endeavor to become very creative with customer acquisition due to our very high responsibility level. You see, we feel that the service we provide is so important to be made available to every single person that requires it, such that we are very aggressive about acquiring customers to their benefit. With this same mindset, customer satisfaction is very high. We are constantly asking patients for feedback and are also constantly asking primary care physician offices for feedback. Staff are expected to have increased responsibility levels as mentioned above, and this translates to decreased amounts of conflict which of course translates to increased longevity with the practice, for the staff that is and the patients.

Calls to office I recorded and reviewed intermittently.

Training of call handling is very important to me. Productivity bonus is linked very strongly to call handling. Staff is given regular feedback about this, and if this improves, staff will be made aware of this, and if this does not improve, they are retrained If this remains a continuous problems despite retraining, then the staff is essentially not allowed to answer the phone, and in fact, his or her time with the company will be terminated unless this is overcome.

Productivity of staff closely linked to a perceived view of patients and primary care physician offices

Production bonus is influenced strongly by feedback from primary care physician offices as well as patients, as already noted. We ask our patients for suggestions as to improving the service they are currently receiving from us and our staff as well as their overall experiences to see how it can be improved upon. Patients are asked for who they recognize highly and are made aware of the fact that we would love to encourage our staff when they need to be encouraged by giving them positive feedback. The converse also applies, if there are any negative recommendations, we ask for the patients to let us know this as well, in which case the staff may have to re-train. This is also done with the primary care physician offices.

Training

Regular training of staff is to make sure of a great experience for the patient and of course, for the primary care physician's office and other vendors that may be doing business with the office. Staff are regularly trained in our offices. There is a weekly meeting with me, every Wednesday, where a training session is done. Staff are trained at weekly meetings, the staff are regularly trained at quarterly meetings with an outside trainer. This is either quarterly or semi-annual. But as you can see, training is paramount, so everyone within the organization continues to improve on their skills, and the ultimate goal of providing the experience for the patient and anyone that interacts with our office that is of value. We are always looking to add value to whoever we impact.

The power of one

With the power of one, the concept is a very strong part of our training and it refers to everyone having a very high responsibility level. In essence, it takes one person and not two people to avoid conflict. It takes one person to create a positive experience as opposed to two people. If one person brings 100% of their game to a relationship expecting 0% in return, there can be no conflict. The highest form or relationship between two human beings is marriage and in marriage if one member of the union brings 100% of themselves to the relationship and expecting 0% in return, the marriage will be a resounding success. Less intimate relationships than this even more so. So with this attitude, the goal is to avoid conflict, and if conflict arises the aim is for the conflict to be resolved very quickly, creating a win-win situation.

Always get a name of who provides service from my office

Getting a name of who provides awesome service is very important both to myself and our staff. It is very important for anyone providing the kind of service I personally want to provide to be recognized, affirmed, and encouraged to continue doing the same or even more. Getting the name of who provides suboptimal service is also very important, because in this case the patient would need to be re-trained. Please always get the name of who provides the service to you, letting me know if it was a positive experience or a negative experience, giving me a chance to be properly represented and correct any inefficiencies in the system. This is something I do all the time in any business I am served by.

This brings us to the end of the sixth chapter. In the next chapter, we'll be talking about the care of the patients by primary care physicians versus nephrologists prior to requiring dialysis.

CHAPTER SEVEN

I can take care of the patients until they are close to requiring dialysis

Utilize the nephrologist to avoid the patient needing dialysis

Alongside your nephrologist prevent and reverse chronic kidney disease progression. This is actually attainable and studies are showing very clearly that the risk factors for chronic kidney disease progression as similar to the risk factors for cardiovascular disease, so lifestyle changes and compliance with this is paramount. This can be done side by side with your nephrologist whom you can use as a resource and you can use to bring some ideas to ultimately provide better service than the service that would have been provided by either one of you. In other words, compliance with care provides increase with both of us on the same page and the patient hearing the same thing from both of us at different times. This way, we reinforce the message and the patient is more apt to comply.

If the patient needs dialysis, mortality is much better if the patient has been followed by a nephrologist for greater than one year prior

This has been proven by very well conducted studies. It is likely because patients tend to be more aware and compliant with treatment if the "specialist" is involved". This likely happens because of the perception by the patient of the seriousness of the condition when the specialist is involved. This fact should be totally exploited such that the patient who hitherto had been non-compliant now deems it necessary to become compliant. Also with more focus care on risk factors, patients are likely to comply and benefit when it is again being reinforced by both care providers.

Do what you do best and let the best do the rest

As a primary care physician, certain things for the patients will be done best by yourself. The things you do best - you do! Anyone else providing care to their patients should reinforce that to the patient and endorse the efforts, absolutely flowing power to you. The things you don't do as well, let the best do. In the current healthcare climate, collaborative care is the way forward and being able to use each other as resources is to each other's benefit, but more importantly to the patient's benefit. Where state-of-the-art evidence based care is offered. It should be better here in the United States than anywhere else in the world.

Morbidity post-dialysis improves if the patient has been seen by a nephrologist greater than one year prior to initiation of dialysis

There is apparently life after dialysis starts. Quality of life is much better if the nephrologist has been involved in the care of the patient for greater than one year prior to initiating dialysis and this has also been proven by very well conducted studies. This is most likely because the nephrologist attempts to be more conscious to avoid muscle and bone loss as a result of attendant metabolic acidosis that occurs in patients with chronic kidney disease. Usually, this occurs as a result of decreased acid secretion into the tubules and decreased bi-carbonate creation by the kidneys.

There is also a stronger focus on the calcium-phosphorus PTH vitamin D axis, which is very important for cardiovascular disease and progression of chronic kidney disease. Preservation of the veins for a possible arteriovenous fistula is also a very important consideration and again, this is a very strong initiative carried out by the nephrologist. The right dialysis modality should be discussed prior to the patient going to stage four of chronic kidney disease. Education has proven to be one of the strongest factors that determines the prognosis of a patient on dialysis, i.e. pre-dialysis education.

We can both take care of patients better than either one of us can alone

Together, we can do much more, i.e. the nephrologist and the primary care physician. On our own independently, we perform a disservice to the patient with chronic kidney disease prior to dialysis. But even more so of course, while on dialysis. Creativity is born from brainstorming. So please brainstorm your patient's care with me. It can only be made better. It definitely will not be made worse.

Modality of dialysis and the time this is discussed and the patient's time-line are big risk factors.

Choosing the right modality as noted above at the right time, is actually very important for patients that will eventually require dialysis. Procedures done for dialysis preparation are more successful if they're done electively. Emergent procedures result in more fistula failure rates and the need for more interventions on the vascular access eventually. Catheter time is a very important concept i.e. decreasing the exposure of the patient on dialysis to intravascular tunneled catheter placements. Continuous dialysis is generally much more physiological and beneficial to the patient in the form of home therapies. Either home hemodialysis or peritoneal dialysis, preferably.

Hospitalizations for non-renal causes improves with the outpatient nephrology consultant continuing to follow in the hospital

Constant follow-up on my patients in the hospital, leads to decreased length of stay in the hospital and decrease morbidity especially as regards to acute kidney injury if I am involved in the patient's care. The rapport that I have with my patient in the out-patient helps provide a comfort and healing mentally, which translates to physical healing while in the hospital. Even though a patient is followed by excellent hospitalists in the hospital, continuity of care with the out-patient specialists involved in their care is more likely if the patient was followed as an in-patient. Numerous surveys have proven this to be the case and even though the patient may be stable, the specialist may follow in a non-active way as there are no other active issues in play.

ENDING CHAPTER

So we have been through seeing the patients in a timely way from referral and then we delved into being able to accept all insurances in the office. After this we tackled providing comprehensive one-stop care for our patients. Followed by discussing the correspondence and how quickly this is received by the primary care physician and then we elaborated on how patients can be cared for by not following up with their primary care physician after seeing a specialist.

Then we discussed the office staff and how easy they are to work with, and finally finished with discussions of the care of patients being done optimally prior to initiation of dialysis. Take action to achieve receiving great feedback from the nephrologist prior to the patient's follow-up, empowering you to provide a great comprehensive follow-up visit for your patient. The first step is to call my office at 407-988-1065 and ask to speak to Ynolandy and tell her, "I want to take advantage of Dr. Awosika's ultimate nephrology body systems and she will get you all set up.